HIGH ALKALINE

DIET

FOR NOVICES

Enriched Recipes, Foods, Meal Plan &
Procedures For Vibrant Health,
Wellness, Prevention Of Cholesterol
And More

DR. MATEO GABRIEL

DISCLAIMER

The information in this book is only meant to be used for general reading. In any way, the author and publisher do not promise or represent that the information in this work is full, correct, reliable, appropriate, or available. This includes any warranties that are expressed or implied. Because of this, you should only rely on this material at your own risk.

This book is not meant to replace professional help. If you have any questions about a subject, you should always get help from a qualified expert. The author and distributor of this book are not responsible for how the information in it is used or abused.

The author's though ts and feelings are shown in this book. They do not necessarily represent the official policy or stance of any other person, group, employer, or business.

Any third-party material that you can get to through this book is not endorsed or backed by the author or publisher.

The information in this book is correct at the time it was published, after all possible checks. However, the author and distributor are not responsible for any loss, damage, or inconvenience that may be caused by mistakes or omissions.

TABLE OF CONTENTS

CHAPTER ONE

INTRODUCTION TO HIGH ALKALINE DIET

THE PH MEASURE

The pH scale, which goes from 0 to 14, indicates how acidic or alkaline a thing is. Neutrality, or a pH of 7, is defined as equilibrium between acidity and alkalinity. Acidity is indicated by values below 7, where lower numbers denote stronger acidity, while alkalinity is shown by values above 7, where higher numbers denote greater alkaline content. Because the scale is logarithmic, a tenfold variation in acidity or alkalinity is represented by each unit. Danish chemist Søren Peder Lauritz

Sørensen first proposed the idea in 1909 as a means of calculating the concentration of hydrogen ions in a solution.

ALKALINE VS. ACIDIC

Fundamental groups having unique properties on the pH scale are acids and bases. Acids are substances with a pH of less than 7, and when they dissolve in water, they release hydrogen ions (H+), which raises the acidity of the solution. Common acids include the hydrochloric acid found in the stomach and the citric acid found in citrus fruits. Conversely, alkaline materials, sometimes referred to as bases, have a pH higher than 7. They cause water to lose some of its acidity by releasing hydroxide ions (OH-). Alkaline materials include soap and baking soda. Acidity and alkalinity must be balanced for several chemical and biological processes to occur.

PH'S FUNCTION IN THE BODY

The human body needs to maintain the right pH balance to function at its best. The body uses a variety of processes, including coordinated efforts between multiple organs and mechanisms, to maintain pH stability. Blood, for example, usually has a pH between 7.35 and 7.45, making it somewhat alkaline. Because even a small change in blood pH can have a significant impact on enzyme activity, cellular function, and other physiological processes, the body closely controls blood pH. The stomach is an exception, though, as it keeps its environment acidic (pH of about 2) to facilitate digestion.

PH is not just important in the stomach and blood. Enzyme activity and food absorption are two examples of cellular functions that are extremely sensitive to pH fluctuations. In addition, a slightly alkaline environment is ideal for the immune system to work. pH imbalances can result in several health problems, depending on the cause diet, stress, or underlying medical diseases. Conditions that impair overall well-being include acidosis (excessive acidity) and alkalosis (excessive alkalinity), which can interfere with cellular function and metabolic functions.

The ability to recognize the delicate balance necessary for good health requires a comprehension of the pH scale, the differences between acidic and alkaline substances, and the function of pH in the body. Sustaining an appropriate pH balance via a nutritious diet, adequate water, and a fit way of life enhances the body's capacity to operate well and fend off potential health problems.

CHAPTER TWO
THE IDEA OF A HIGH ALKALINE DIET
MEANING AND FOUNDATIONS

The core tenet of the high-alkaline diet concept is that general health and well-being can be enhanced by keeping the body's pH level slightly alkaline. The foundation of this dietary strategy is the idea that eating foods that generate an alkaline state helps balance out the acidity that results from eating a diet high in processed foods, sugar, and animal products. The basic idea is that people can improve several physiological processes, lessen inflammation, and possibly even minimize their chance of developing chronic diseases by maintaining a pH balance in their bodies.

AN HISTORICAL ANGLE

The idea of an alkaline diet originated in ancient medicine when some societies stressed the significance of keeping the body's acidity and alkalinity in balance. For example, Ayurveda and traditional Chinese medicine have long acknowledged the role that nutrition plays in maintaining health and preventing illness. However, the work of scientists and medical professionals who investigated how diet affected the body's acid-base balance is largely responsible for the modern interpretation of the alkaline diet's rise to prominence in the early 20th century.

ADVANTAGES OF AN ALKALINE DIET

Supporters of the alkaline diet point to the diet's ability to bolster the body's innate systems for preserving health as one of its main advantages. Proponents contend that eating foods high in alkali, like fruits, vegetables, and some grains, helps people establish a body environment that makes the body less prone to inflammation and illness. Additionally, some proponents assert that an alkaline diet might boost vitality overall, assist in weight loss, and increase energy levels.

Furthermore, the alkaline diet is frequently linked to the idea that it could aid in the prevention or treatment of several medical disorders, such as osteoporosis. It is hypothesized that maintaining bone density can be achieved by decreasing the body's need for calcium dissolved from bones to counteract excessive acidity through a diet high in alkaline-forming foods. Although there is conflicting scientific information about the direct link between dietary acidity and osteoporosis, the alkaline diet is frequently advocated as a prophylactic against problems relating to the bones.

Moreover, proponents of the alkaline diet assert that it could extend life and offer anti-aging benefits. They contend that inflammation and oxidative stress, which are thought to speed up aging, can be mitigated by eating foods that generate an alkaline environment. It's crucial to remember that there is little scientific proof for these assertions, and more research is needed.

The High Alkaline Diet Concept is predicated on the notion that eating foods that generate an alkaline environment and keeping the body's pH at a slightly alkaline level can have several positive health effects. Traditional medicine has historical perspectives on the body's acidity and alkalinity balance, but the modern interpretation rose to prominence in the

20th century. Proponents highlight possible advantages including anti-aging properties, improved energy, support for bone health, and less inflammation. Though the scientific evidence for some of these claims is still developing, it is important to approach these claims with a skeptical mentality.

CHAPTER THREE

THE BODY'S SYSTEMS FOR REGULATING PH

ACID-BASE BALANCE AND THE KIDNEYS

The maintenance of homeostasis, which guarantees the best possible functioning of physiological processes, depends critically on the regulation of the body's pH. The kidneys are one of the main participants in this control since they are essential in preserving the acid-base balance. In reaction to changes in blood pH, the kidneys accomplish this by excreting hydrogen ions and selectively reabsorbing bicarbonate ions.

This renal process is critical for maintaining long-term pH balance and preventing the body from becoming overly acidic or alkaline.

ROLE OF THE RESPIRATORY SYSTEM

On the other hand, the respiratory system makes a substantial contribution to the body's ability to maintain its pH levels. The respiratory system aids in controlling the amount of bicarbonate ions in the blood by removing carbon dioxide (CO_2) through the lungs. Carbonic anhydrase is the enzyme that catalyzes the reaction between CO_2 and water to generate carbonic acid. The respiratory rate regulates the body's ability to eliminate CO_2, which in turn affects the amounts of bicarbonate and carbonic acid ions and, ultimately, pH.

BODY'S BUFFER SYSTEMS

The body's buffer systems, which absorb or release hydrogen ions, play a critical role in preventing significant pH fluctuations. One of the main extracellular buffer systems that keeps blood plasma at a constant pH is the bicarbonate buffer system. The kidneys and lungs are responsible for maintaining the equilibrium between bicarbonate ions and carbonic acid in this system. The phosphate buffer system helps maintain the ideal pH range for biological functions inside cells by aiding in intracellular pH regulation.

Hemoglobin in particular is one of the key intracellular buffers that proteins play. The histidine residues in hemoglobin can either take in or release protons, which helps red blood cells buffer. Furthermore, by interacting with hydrogen ions, proteins in the blood help resist pH shifts. These buffer systems must operate efficiently to prevent abrupt changes in pH that can be harmful to enzyme activity and general cellular health.

CHAPTER FOUR

ESSENTIALS OF AN ALKALINE DIET

FOODS HIGH IN ALKALI AND PH LEVELS

The alkaline diet concept is centered on food pH levels and how they affect the body's overall acidity. Potential hydrogen, or pH, is a scale that goes from 0 to 14 that indicates how acidic or alkaline a substance is. A pH of seven is regarded as neutral; values that are lower or higher than seven denote acidity or alkalinity, respectively. Foods classified as alkaline have a pH of greater than 7, and individuals who follow the alkaline diet contend that eating a larger percentage of these foods can help keep the body's environment more alkaline. Commonly consumed alkaline foods include beans, nuts, fruits, and vegetables; these foods are thought to support a more balanced pH level within the body.

ACIDIC VS. ALKALINE FOODS

Within the framework of the alkaline diet, foods are frequently classified as acidic or alkaline according to how they affect the pH levels of the body. As previously stated, meals that are alkaline have a pH of more than 7, whereas those that are acidic have a pH of less than 7. The alkaline diet's proponents assert that eating a diet high in alkaline foods can help mitigate the negative effects of the typical Western diet, which is high in acidic items including meat, dairy, processed foods, and refined carbohydrates. The idea is to tip the scales in favor of more alkaline meals to create an internally alkaline environment that is thought to boost general health and well-being.

MAKING AN OPTIMAL ALKALINE PLATE

Choosing a range of alkaline foods to create a balanced and nutrient-dense meal is the first step in creating an alkaline-optimized plate. Fresh fruits and vegetables—especially those with a high alkaline content—should be included. Broccoli, avocados, cucumbers, and leafy greens are frequently suggested as foundational foods for an alkaline-optimized diet. Apart from veggies, a well-rounded diet can also include alkaline grains like quinoa and millet, as well as alkaline-forming proteins like tofu and other legumes. To preserve the appropriate pH balance, proponents of the alkaline diet also advise minimizing or staying away from acidic items like dairy, red meat, and processed meals.

ALKALINE MEAL PLANS EXAMPLE

A variety of nutrient-dense foods are included in sample alkaline meal plans to guarantee a balance of vital vitamins and minerals. A meal plan might call for a green smoothie composed of spinach, kale, and berries, which are alkaline-forming foods, for breakfast. A quinoa salad with an abundance of vibrant greens and avocado on top for extra alkalinity may be the meal. Dinner could be alkaline-focused, such as roasted veggies on the side and grilled tofu. Nuts, seeds, and fresh fruits are examples of snack foods. It is noteworthy that the nutritional requirements of individuals differ, and seeking advice from a healthcare practitioner or a qualified nutritionist is recommended when making substantial dietary modifications.

The alkaline diet is based on the idea that eating foods high in acidity can help the body's pH levels to balance. Creating well-rounded, alkaline-optimized plates and knowing the difference between acidic and alkaline meals might be important parts of following this dietary strategy.

CHAPTER FIVE
THE NEED FOR HYDRATION
PH-NEUTRAL WATER

Drinking alkaline water is one of the hottest ideas when it comes to staying hydrated. Alkaline water proponents contend that by balancing the body's pH levels, they can improve general health. Alkaline water is said to be able to balance acidic elements in the body and usually has a higher pH than ordinary tap water. Although there is little scientific proof to back up these claims, some people swear by the health advantages of alkaline water and highlight its potential to support optimal health.

ADVANTAGES OF ADEQUATE HYDRATION

It is impossible to exaggerate how important staying hydrated is to preserving general health. Drinking enough water is essential for several body processes, such as regulating body temperature, moving nutrients through the body, and lubricating joints. Consuming enough water also improves focus and concentration by supporting cognitive function. Furthermore, maintaining adequate fluid balance is essential for the functioning of critical organs like the kidneys, which depend on them for normal function. All things considered, preserving ideal levels of hydration plays a major role in the body's capacity to carry out several physiological processes.

DIY RECIPES FOR ALKALINE WATER

There are several homemade recipes for alkaline water that people can use as part of their daily hydration regimen. Adding flavors to water, such as lemon, cucumber, and mint, is one common technique. It is thought that these components contain alkalizing qualities, which could raise the pH of the water.

These recipes provide a tasty and refreshing substitute for regular water, even if they might not significantly change the pH of the liquid. It's important to remember that the evidence supporting the possible health advantages of homemade alkaline water recipes is still mostly anecdotal, so speaking with a healthcare provider is advised.

HEALTHY ALKALINE FOODS

Apart from alkaline water, some foods are also labeled as "alkaline superfoods" because they are thought to support the preservation or restoration of the body's ideal pH balance. Due to their high mineral content, which includes potassium and magnesium, green leafy vegetables are frequently included in this group. It is believed that these minerals have alkalizing properties for the body. Alkaline-forming foods include nuts and seeds, which provide necessary nutrients and may also help balance acidity. Although adding alkaline superfoods to the diet can have several positive health effects, it's important to keep your diet varied and well-balanced overall.

LEAFY GREEN VEGETABLES

Vegetables that are rich in vitamins, minerals, and antioxidants are considered nutritional powerhouses. These veggies, which range from collard greens and Swiss chard to kale and spinach, have numerous health advantages. Their high water content is significant when it comes to hydration. Eating leafy green veggies increases nutritional intake overall and helps with hydration. Water and vital nutrients support body processes and contribute to optimum health maintenance.

ACIDIC FRUITS

Some fruits are considered to be beneficial contributions to a well-balanced diet because of their alkalizing qualities. Watermelon, lemons, and limes are a few examples. These fruits have an acidic taste at first, but they metabolize in a way that is thought to produce an alkaline effect on the body. Alkaline fruits are high in water content, which helps to hydrate the body. They also include important vitamins and antioxidants that support general health and well-being.

SEEDS AND NUTS

Nuts and seeds are adaptable supplements to a well-balanced diet, providing a blend of necessary nutrients, protein, and healthy fats. These foods, which include flaxseeds, chia seeds, and walnuts, are regarded as alkaline-forming. Even while they might not have as much moisture as fruits and vegetables, their alkalizing properties make them useful additions to a diet that aims to keep the body's pH balance in check. Adding a range of nuts and seeds to one's diet enhances overall nutritional diversity as well as hydration.

CHAPTER SIX

HOW TO ADOPT A HIGH ALKALINE DIET

CHANGING YOUR LIFESTYLE TO AN ALKALINE ONE

A substantial change in eating habits and way of life is required when starting the High Alkaline Diet. The foundation of this eating strategy is the notion that the body can prevent and improve overall health by keeping its pH at a slightly alkaline level. A careful and educated strategy is needed to make the switch to an alkaline lifestyle, taking into account daily activities, personal preferences, and health issues.

It entails adopting a diet that is mostly plant-based and consuming fewer acidic foods.

MODEST VS. QUICK CHANGES

Selecting whether to make quick or gradual dietary changes is an important part of following the High Alkaline Diet. By easing the body into the new eating patterns gradually, gradual modifications provide a more tolerable transition and minimize the risk of adverse effects. With this method, the consumption of acidic meals is gradually reduced while alkaline-rich foods including fruits, vegetables, and nuts are gradually added. Conversely, other people could want to make quick adjustments and adopt an alkaline lifestyle more quickly. Although this can produce benefits more quickly, there may be difficulties as the body can require some time to adjust to such a significant change.

OVERCOMING OBSTACLES

Adopting an alkaline lifestyle has its share of difficulties. Making the switch to a plant-based diet can be challenging, particularly for people who are used to an acidic or processed diet. To overcome this obstacle, try experimenting with different alkaline foods, learn new recipes, and find fun substitutes for your favorite acidic foods.

Furthermore, social situations including a lot of acidic foods may need to be planned and communicated with. The key to overcoming the difficulties of following the High Alkaline Diet is to remain steadfast and driven in the face of temptation.

ADVICE FOR PROLONGED ACHIEVEMENT

To sustain an alkaline lifestyle over the long run, a supportive environment, lifestyle modifications, and mindful eating are all necessary. A diet rich in nutrients and well-balanced is ensured by including a wide variety of alkaline foods. Overall success is influenced by preparing meals in advance, drinking alkaline water to stay hydrated, and implementing alkaline-promoting behaviors like frequent exercise and stress reduction. Creating a network of support or consulting with doctors, dietitians, or other healthcare providers can offer insightful advice and motivation for long-term High Alkaline Diet adherence.

Whether one chooses a gradual or immediate method, making the switch to an alkaline lifestyle demands careful thought. Success requires overcoming obstacles, such as transitioning to a plant-based diet and interacting with others. People should concentrate on creating a supportive atmosphere, making lifestyle changes, and practicing mindful eating to sustain long-term adherence. One can take advantage of the High Alkaline Diet's potential advantages for general health and well-being by adopting these ideas.

CHAPTER SEVEN

THE ALKALINE DIET AND MANAGING WEIGHT

THE ALKALINE DIET AND MANAGING WEIGHT

The foundation of the alkaline diet is the idea that eating foods that promote alkaline balance can have a good effect on both managing weight and general health. This diet strategy revolves around the idea of alkalinity and how it could affect metabolism. A substance's alkalinity is determined by its pH level; a value of 7 or more is regarded as alkaline. The Alkaline Diet's proponents contend that by keeping the body's pH slightly alkaline, metabolic processes can be improved and nutrients can be used for energy production more effectively.

METABOLISM AND ALKALINITY

The intricate system of chemical processes known as metabolism is essential for maintaining a healthy weight. According to the Alkaline Diet, an alkaline environment promotes metabolic processes, which may improve the body's capacity to metabolize food and turn it into energy. Because of this supposed connection between metabolism and alkalinity, some people have started using the Alkaline Diet as a weight-loss plan.

IMPACTS ON LOSING WEIGHT

The Alkaline Diet's apparent impact on weight loss is one of its noteworthy side effects. Proponents contend that people can induce fat loss by focusing on meals that are high in alkalinity, such as fruits, vegetables, and some grains. The reasoning behind this is that an alkaline state may encourage the breakdown of excess fat in the body, whilst an acidic state may cause it to be stored. It's crucial to remember that there is little scientific proof to back up these particular assertions and that each person's reaction to the diet will be different.

INCREASING MUSCLE LEANNESS

Moreover, the impact of the Alkaline Diet on weight control goes beyond weight reduction. It is frequently proposed that this dietary strategy promotes the development of lean muscle mass. The focus on alkaline-forming, plant-based diets offers a nutrient-rich base that promotes the growth and repair of muscles. An adequate amount of protein, which is essential for developing muscle, can be obtained from plant-based sources including nuts, seeds, and legumes—all of which are mainstays of the Alkaline Diet. Not only is gaining lean muscle mass necessary for a toned body, but it also raises basal metabolic rate, which may help with long-term weight control.

Finally, the Alkaline Diet suggests a link between metabolism, alkalinity, and controlling weight. Although there is evidence that an alkaline environment may benefit various areas of health, it is best to proceed cautiously when it comes to particular claims about lean muscle mass and weight loss. The efficacy of any dietary strategy is dependent on a variety of factors, including personal preferences, desires, and requirements.

CHAPTER EIGHT

ALKALINE DIET AND PARTICULAR MEDICAL DISORDERS

DIGESTIVE HEALTH AND ACID REFLUX

The Alkaline Diet has drawn interest due to its possible advantages in treating acid reflux and enhancing digestive health in general. When stomach acid refluxes back into the esophagus, it can be uncomfortable and irritating. The alkaline diet's proponents contend that by bringing the body's pH levels into balance, it can aid in symptom relief. The diet discourages the consumption of acidic foods like coffee, processed meals, and some meats and promotes the consumption of alkaline-forming foods like fruits, vegetables, and certain grains.

This method is justified by the idea that digestive problems may be exacerbated by an acidic internal environment. It is believed that foods that generate an alkaline environment balance out too much acidity. Although there isn't much scientific proof to directly link the Alkaline Diet to acid reflux, some research indicates that eating a lot of fruits and vegetables may be good for digestive health. But to receive individualized guidance catered to their particular requirements, those suffering from acid reflux must speak with medical professionals.

OSTEOPENIA AND BONE HEALTH

There has been discussion about the possible connection between osteoporosis and the Alkaline Diet and bone health. Weakened and brittle bones are a hallmark of osteoporosis, which increases a person's risk of fractures. The Alkaline Diet's proponents contend that by keeping the body's pH slightly alkaline, eating foods that are alkaline-forming may improve bone health.

It is thought that some acidic foods encourage the loss of calcium from the bones, which lowers bone density. The Alkaline Diet seeks to prevent this possible calcium loss and promote bone health by placing a strong emphasis on fruits, vegetables, and low-acid grains. Yet, there is conflicting scientific evidence to back up these assertions, and the relationship between dietary pH and bone health is complicated and involves several interrelated elements.

Although eating a diet high in fruits and vegetables is generally linked to better health outcomes, it's important to take into account other factors that may affect bone health, like overall nutrition, hormone balance, and physical activity. People who are worried about osteoporosis should speak with medical professionals to create a complete bone health plan that includes a healthy diet, regular exercise, and supplements if needed.

FOR CHRONIC INFLAMMATION, AN ALKALINE DIET

Numerous medical problems, such as autoimmune illnesses, diabetes, and cardiovascular disease, are frequently associated with chronic inflammation. The Alkaline Diet is a dietary strategy that promotes an alkaline state in the body, which is thought to reduce inflammation. Proponents contend that by counteracting excessive acidity and fostering an alkaline atmosphere, foods that are alkaline-forming can aid in the reduction of inflammation.

Alkaline diet mainstays, fruits, and vegetables, are abundant in anti-inflammatory substances including phytochemicals and antioxidants. Although these foods may have anti-inflammatory qualities and can improve general health, research on how the Alkaline Diet directly affects chronic inflammation is still ongoing.

CHAPTER NINE

MONITORING AND TESTING FOR PH

METHODS FOR HOME PH TESTING

For people who wish to keep an eye on the acidity or alkalinity of different substances in their living space, at-home pH testing devices are indispensable. Assessing the quality of the water is one situation where pH testing at home is frequently used. A lot of people assess the pH of their aquariums or drinking water using pH testing kits. Usually, these kits come with liquid reagents that change color according to the pH level or pH test strips.

After that, the color shift is interpreted by comparing it to a comparable pH scale.

Soil analysis for gardening purposes is another common use for pH testing at home. Knowing the pH of the soil enables gardeners to choose the right plants to grow and the additions that will help them grow to their full potential. Different plants like different pH ranges. To measure the acidity or alkalinity of the soil with accuracy, home gardeners frequently utilize soil pH meters or pH testing probes.

ANALYZING PH FINDINGS

Since it sheds light on the characteristics of the material being examined, interpreting pH test findings is an essential part of the process. Seven is regarded as neutral on the pH scale, which goes from 0 to 14. Something is acidic if its pH is less than 7, and basic or alkaline if its pH is greater than 7. Greater alkalinity is suggested by a higher pH, whilst greater acidity is indicated by a lower pH. In a variety of situations, knowing a substance's pH level is essential. For instance, the efficacy of pool chemicals and swimmer comfort both depend on the water's pH being maintained at the right level.

When it comes to drinking water, a pH of 6.5 to 8.5 is usually regarded as acceptable for human consumption. Variations outside of this range, however, may have an impact on flavor, pipe corrosion, and the effectiveness of water treatment procedures. Because different kinds of aquatic life have varying pH preferences, aquarium enthusiasts also rely on pH testing to establish an appropriate habitat for fish and other aquatic life.

FREQUENCY OF EXAMINATION

The type of substance being tested and its significance in a given situation determines how frequently a substance is tested for pH. For example, householders can test the pH of their drinking water sources regularly to make sure the water quality is maintained. On the other hand, gardeners may check the pH of the soil more often, particularly after adding soil additives or after introducing new plants. Hobbyists who own aquariums may periodically test the pH of their tanks because variations can affect the well-being of the aquatic life.

Testing pH levels regularly is especially crucial for systems like hydroponic gardens or swimming pools where pH is crucial. In these situations, the system's overall performance and functionality depend on keeping a constant pH level. Testing frequency is generally dictated by various criteria, including past pH-related problems, drug origin, and consumption habits.

Home pH testing kits are useful instruments for keeping an eye on and preserving the pH values of different materials in our living spaces. Decisions on ideal conditions are guided by the interpretation of pH data, which offers insights into the nature of the chemical being examined. The context and the significance of preserving a particular pH range for the intended results determine how frequently pH tests should be conducted. pH testing is an adaptable technique with applications in a variety of contexts, including guaranteeing safe drinking water, encouraging plant growth, and establishing an appropriate environment for aquatic life.

CHAPTER TEN
ALKALINE DIET AND PREVENTIVE MEDICINE
CANCER PREVENTION

In recent years, there has been interest in and research on the connection between the alkaline diet and cancer prevention. The alkaline diet's proponents contend that keeping the body's pH slightly alkaline can reduce the conditions that encourage the development and spread of cancer cells. According to the notion, an acidic environment may exacerbate inflammation and weaken the immune system, which could lead to the onset of cancer. It's crucial to remember that there is scant and equivocal scientific data to back up these assertions.

The main focus of research on the alkaline diet's ability to prevent cancer is on how alkaline foods, like fruits and vegetables, may be able to lower oxidative stress and inflammation. Antioxidants and other phytochemicals found in abundance in these foods may offer protection against specific cancer types. Although an alkaline diet by itself cannot be regarded as a foolproof method of preventing cancer, including a range of alkaline-promoting foods in a healthy and well-balanced diet may improve general health and maybe reduce the risk of cancer.

CARDIOVASCULAR HEALTH

Because fruits, vegetables, and other plant-based foods are known to have heart-protective qualities, the alkaline diet has a connection to cardiovascular health. Due to their generally low cholesterol and saturated fat content, these meals help to maintain normal blood lipid profiles and lower the risk of cardiovascular illnesses. A diet high in foods that promote alkaline digestion may also aid in blood pressure regulation and enhance endothelial function.

According to studies, an alkaline diet that is rich in fruits and vegetables can reduce the risk of cardiovascular disease by reducing oxidative stress, inflammation, and arterial stiffness. Because they help regulate blood pressure, alkaline minerals like potassium found in these foods also contribute to cardiovascular health. But rather than concentrating just on food pH, it's important to take lifestyle and general dietary patterns into account.

DIABETES MANAGEMENT

The alkaline diet may be beneficial for those who are managing their diabetes. Fresh fruits and vegetables are among the nutrient-dense, low-glycemic foods that are encouraged in the diet because they can help control blood sugar levels. These foods lower the risk of severe blood sugar rises and crashes by releasing glucose into the system gradually.

Furthermore, the alkaline diet's emphasis on staying away from highly refined and processed foods is consistent with standard advice for managing diabetes. Processed foods frequently include refined carbs and added sugars, which can worsen blood sugar regulation and lead to insulin resistance. The alkaline diet may supplement diabetes management efforts by encouraging a whole-food, plant-based approach; nonetheless, individuals with diabetes must collaborate with healthcare providers to develop a customized, well-balanced dietary plan.

Even if the alkaline diet may be beneficial for managing diabetes, preventing cancer, and improving cardiovascular health, it is important to approach these claims cautiously and take into account the larger context of general dietary patterns and lifestyle factors. Making educated decisions about illness prevention and management still requires speaking with medical experts and depending on evidence-based procedures.

CHAPTER ELEVEN

DISPELLING OFTEN HELD MYTHS

MYTHS ABOUT THE ALKALINE DIET

Proponents of the alkaline diet claim that eating foods that create an alkaline environment can improve health and prevent several illnesses, which has led to the diet's rise in popularity. There are, however, a few myths regarding this nutritional strategy. A common misconception is that the body's pH levels can be directly impacted by an alkaline diet. The pH balance of the human body is very closely regulated, and dietary modifications have little effect on this sensitive balance. Urine pH can be influenced by specific diets, but this is not a good measure of how acidic the body is generally.

Another prevalent misperception is the idea that all foods high in acidity are unhealthy and therefore to be avoided. Foods are classified as acidic or alkaline according to the amount of ash left over after digestion in the alkaline diet. Nevertheless, there is no guarantee that this classification will correspond with the food's pH before eating or its health effects. Citrus fruits, for instance, despite being classified as acidic, their mineral content can have alkalizing effects on the body.

SCIENTIFIC REBUTTALS

The alkaline diet's detractors contend that there is little scientific data to support its theoretical claims. Although specific eating patterns may impact the acid-base balance, advocates of the alkaline diet tend to oversimplify their broader arguments. The kidneys and lungs are two of the body's buffering systems that are essential for preserving pH homeostasis, which limits the effects of dietary changes.

Moreover, the alkaline diet oversimplifies the complexity of nutrition by emphasizing certain food groups. Numerous health benefits of eating a diversified, balanced diet high in fruits, vegetables, and whole grains have been shown by scientific studies. Still, it is simplistic to attribute these advantages to the alkalinity of individual meals and ignore the complex interactions between various nutrients and chemicals found in a varied diet.

DEALING WITH SKEPTICISM

It is crucial to promote a critical analysis of the existing data to dispel doubt about the alkaline diet. Alkaline diet proponents frequently mention anecdotal success stories, but they are not the same as scientific evidence. Examining peer-reviewed studies that look into how nutrition affects health outcomes is a more rigorous method.

Furthermore, it is imperative to recognize that individual responses to diets differ. Health consequences are influenced by a variety of factors, including lifestyle, heredity, and general food habits. Opponents contend that rather than strictly following an alkaline diet, which can cause nutritional imbalances, the emphasis should be on encouraging a balanced and nutrient-dense diet.

Dispelling widespread misconceptions about the alkaline diet necessitates a sophisticated comprehension of how the body regulates pH, a critical assessment of the available data, and an appreciation of the complexity of nutrition. Although the alkaline diet may have some elements that are consistent with basic health-conscious eating guidelines, one should proceed cautiously when dealing with inflated claims and simplistic categorizations.

CHAPTER TWELVE

WORKING OUT AND ALKALINITY

EXERCISE'S EFFECT ON PH

The body's pH levels are significantly affected by exercise, which also affects the delicate balance between acidity and alkalinity. Lactic acid is one of the byproducts that are produced by the metabolic processes in the muscles during physical activity. These metabolites may cause an acidic spike that lasts just a short while, which lowers pH levels. This is sometimes referred to as exercise-induced acidosis.

Nonetheless, the body has systems in place to control pH levels both before and after exercise. The respiratory system is one such process that aids in the removal of surplus carbon dioxide, another acidic consequence of metabolism. Body fluids, including blood, also have a buffering capacity that helps to keep the pH at a somewhat steady level. Exercise regularly can improve the effectiveness of these regulating systems, which in turn improves the acid-base balance.

TOP ALKALINE-FRIENDLY EXERCISE PLANS

Some exercise regimens are thought to be more alkaline-friendly, encouraging the body to have a balanced pH environment. Running, swimming, and cycling are examples of aerobic workouts that are well-known for improving oxygen use and lowering lactic acid generation. By fostering an atmosphere that is better suited to preserving alkalinity, these activities reduce the possibility of exercise-induced acidosis.

Yoga and other low-impact exercises are beneficial for fostering alkalinity as well. These practices emphasize deliberate movement and regulated breathing, which helps soothe the nervous system. Stress-related acidity can be reduced by emphasizing relaxation and appropriate breathing, which promotes an alkaline internal environment.

MANAGING SLEEP AND EXERCISE

Maintaining the body's ideal pH levels requires striking a balance between rest and exercise. Exercise is good for your health in general, but if you exercise too much without getting enough rest, you may accumulate acidic byproducts. The body can heal and rebuild during rest and recovery times, which helps to promote the removal of metabolic waste and delay the onset of acidosis.

Getting enough sleep is just as important to a fitness regimen as doing the exercises.

This equilibrium becomes especially crucial for sportsmen and fitness fanatics who follow rigorous training schedules. The body can regulate acidity and maintain a more alkaline condition when it gets enough sleep, drinks enough water, and engages in mindful healing techniques.

Physical activity affects pH levels dynamically and can cause a brief shift in the body's pH toward acidity. However, maintaining a good pH balance is aided by the body's natural regulatory mechanisms, particular exercise regimens, and a balanced attitude to rest and activity.

CHAPTER THIRTEEN

RECIPES FOR ALKALINE BREAKFASTS

INVIGORATING DRINKS

Smoothies are a well-liked option for individuals looking for an alkaline and nutrient-rich breakfast. These colorful mixtures usually contain a range of alkaline fruits and vegetables, which are great sources of vitamins and minerals and also help maintain the pH balance of the body. Leafy greens like spinach or kale, as well as alkaline fruits like kiwi, berries, and citrus fruits, are common ingredients. People can also add alkaline water or a little lemon juice to their smoothies to increase the alkalinity. The blend of these alkaline components not only results in a tasty and refreshing morning drink but also gives you a natural energy boost to start the day.

ALKALINE BREAKFAST BOWLS WITH OATMEAL

For individuals who would like to have a more conventional start to the day, alkaline oatmeal and breakfast bowls provide a filling and substantial alternative. Because they contain mildly alkaline oats, these bowls offer a balanced and nutrient-dense breakfast option when paired with alkaline-rich toppings. In addition to adding taste and texture, ingredients like sliced bananas, almonds, chia seeds, and a drizzle of coconut milk help make the meal more alkaline. Because it contains whole grains and alkaline-rich toppings, it provides a steady energy release throughout the morning, which makes it a great option for people who lead active lives or who want to stick to an alkaline-focused diet.

IDEAS FOR BREAKFAST SALADS

Despite their unusual appearance, breakfast salads provide a nutrient-rich and refreshing substitute for more conventional morning meals. Alkaline veggies, leafy greens, and protein sources like quinoa or tofu are frequently combined in these salads. Cucumbers, tomatoes, avocados, and bell peppers are a few examples of ingredients that add color and provide a variety of vitamins and minerals. Light vinaigrette made with alkaline-friendly ingredients like olive oil and apple cider vinegar can be poured over the greens to increase the alkalinity of the salad. As a consequence, you have a breakfast salad that tastes great and gives you the energy and lightness you need to take on the day.

CHAPTER THIRTEEN

ALKALINE RECIPES FOR LUNCH AND DINNER

PLANT-BASED MAIN COURSES

In line with the tenets of an alkaline diet, which stress the consumption of nutrient-dense, alkaline-forming foods, plant-based main courses are an essential part of alkaline lunch and dinner recipes. Legumes, whole grains, and vegetables are among the many plant-based components that are primarily included in these main dishes. Among the mainstays are quinoa, kale, chickpeas, and lentils; these serve as the basis for a wide variety of recipes that suit various tastes.

Quinoa and black bean bowls are a common main course made of alkaline plants. Complete protein quinoa goes well with black beans to create a filling and healthy dinner. Avocado, cherry tomatoes, and colorful bell peppers add vital vitamins and minerals in addition to improving the dish's aesthetic appeal. This recipe is a great example of how the alkaline diet stresses the importance of including a range of colorful, plant-based elements.

ALKALINE SOUPS AND STEWS

For individuals following an alkaline diet, alkaline soups and stews provide a warming and nourishing alternative. These recipes usually include a variety of legumes and vegetables that generate an alkaline environment, resulting in a tasty broth. Lentils, spinach, broccoli, and carrots are a few examples of items found in a traditional alkaline soup. These ingredients are high in vitamins, minerals, and fiber in addition to adding to the dish's alkalinity.

Alkaline-promoting herbs and spices like turmeric, ginger, and garlic frequently contribute to the alkaline quality of these soups and stews. Along with improving the flavor profile, some substances have added health benefits, such as antioxidant and anti-inflammatory qualities. Thus, alkaline soups and stews offer a comprehensive strategy for enhancing well-being via a balanced diet.

Alkaline lunch and dinner recipes revolve around satisfying salads, which offer a tasty and revitalizing approach to include items that form an alkaline diet. Leafy greens, a variety of vibrant veggies, and alkaline-rich components define these salads. To create a pleasing balance of flavors and textures, kale, arugula, cherry tomatoes, cucumber, and avocado can all be combined in a traditional alkaline salad.

Dressings with a lemon or lime basis are usually chosen over acidic ones to bring out the alkaline qualities of the salad. Alkaline-forming seeds and nuts, like pumpkin seeds or almonds, improve the nutritional profile and give the dish a pleasing crunch. In addition to being in line with the principles of the alkaline diet, satisfying salads offer a wide range of nutrients that promote general health and well-being.

A dedication to the fundamentals of the alkaline diet is demonstrated by the inclusion of plant-based main courses, satisfying salads, and alkaline soups and stews in regular meals.

CHAPTER FOURTEEN

ALKALINE DESSERTS AND SNACKS

SNACKS HIGH IN NUTRIENTS

When it comes to alkaline snacks, choosing nutrient-dense selections is essential for promoting general well-being. A range of fruits, vegetables, nuts, and seeds are commonly included in these snacks, all of which provide important vitamins, minerals, and antioxidants. Cucumbers and bell peppers are two great examples of raw veggies that go well with hummus or guacamole because they add a nice crunch and extra nutrients. In addition to being delicious, fresh fruits like apples, watermelon, and berries also produce alkaline bodies, which support a pH equilibrium within the body.

Nuts and seeds are excellent additions to your arsenal of alkaline snacks. Nutritious fats, fiber, and an abundance of vitamins and minerals may be found in almonds, walnuts, chia seeds, and flaxseeds. Combining these nuts and seeds to make a trail mix guarantees a varied nutrient intake while adding appeal. Furthermore, adding alkaline-forming grains to snacks, such as buckwheat or quinoa, can offer a prolonged energy release, which makes them a great option for people looking for a balanced diet.

NO-GUILT ALKALINE DESSERTS

Accepting guilt-free alkaline desserts enables people to satisfy their sweet tooths without sacrificing their health. A popular option is avocado-based chocolate mousse, which combines the rich flavor of cocoa with the creamy texture of avocado. In addition to being tasty, this dish forms an alkaline environment because it is sweetened with natural sweeteners like agave or maple syrup. Berry parfaits are a lovely dessert that is visually appealing and nutritional. They are made with layers of fresh berries, coconut yogurt, and a sprinkle of alkaline-forming nuts or seeds.

Nut flour and coconut flour can also be used in place of conventional refined flour in alkaline dessert recipes. This replacement offers a gluten-free option in addition to preserving the alkaline balance. Raw sweets are easy, filling choices that pack a sweet punch without the guilt, like these no-bake energy balls with coconut, almonds, and dates. The secret is to choose components that will satisfy your sweet needs while adhering to the principles of the alkaline diet.

DRINKS THAT REHYDRATE

Drinks are vital for keeping things in balance when it comes to alkaline hydration. Alkaline fruit juices, such as lime or lemon, can be added fresh to water to improve its flavor and alkalinity. Herbal teas are a calming and hydrating choice, especially when mixed with alkaline-forming herbs like peppermint or dandelion. In addition to being a nutrient-dense snack, alkaline-rich leafy greens, cucumber, and celery make up a green smoothie.

Because of its high electrolyte content, coconut water is a hydrating beverage that is compatible with an alkaline diet. It supplies necessary minerals in addition to quenching thirst, promoting an overall alkaline balance. Alkaline fruits, such as watermelon or berries, have a high nutrient profile and taste, which makes water more palatable and encourages drinking more of it. The key to maintaining the body's natural pH balance and fostering maximum health is drinking plenty of alkaline water.